CHAIR YOGA FOR SENIORS OVER 60

Improve Flexibility, Boost Strength, and
Enhance Well-Being with Gentle,
Easy-to-Follow Chair Yoga Routines
Designed for Seniors

James Deck

Table Of Content

1

Introduction

An easy and low-impact exercise regimen, chair yoga is beneficial for seniors over 60. Chair yoga, as opposed to traditional yoga, uses a chair as a prop for support, making it easier for persons who struggle with balance, mobility, or joint pain to practice. It is a moderate strategy that offers numerous physical, mental, and emotional advantages for seniors looking to maintain or improve their overall well-being.

The Advantages of Senior Chair Yoga

Seniors who practice chair yoga might get many benefits. Greater flexibility is among the most important benefits. Our range of motion is limited as we age because our muscles and joints begin to stiffen. With the gentle stretching provided by chair yoga, seniors can preserve or even regain flexibility without running the danger of strain. The deliberate and deliberate motions target various muscle areas to promote increased range of motion.

Chair yoga not only increases flexibility but also muscle strength. Aging causes many elders to lose muscle, which reduces their strength and stability. Exercises in chair yoga focus on the arms, legs, and core in particular, which helps to develop strength in a supported and safe way. A typical worry among seniors is falling, however this improvement in muscular tone can help with general balance and lower the risk of falling.

In addition, chair yoga lowers stress and improves mental clarity. Yoga's mindfulness and breathing exercises serve to ease the mind, lessen anxiety, and enhance concentration. Chair yoga can help seniors feel more in control of their stress levels and improve their mental wellbeing. Seniors may feel overburdened by the responsibilities of aging or long-term medical concerns.

How Doing Chair Yoga Can Enhance Your Life Quality

Chair yoga is essential for improving your general quality of life in addition to your physical wellness. Regular physical activity enhances energy levels, lessens arthritic pain, and improves circulation. A regular chair yoga practice helps many seniors sleep better, feel less tense physically, and have more energy throughout the day.

Additionally, chair yoga promotes a feeling of connection and community. Taking chair yoga classes, whether in person or virtually, can help seniors overcome feelings of isolation and loneliness by giving them a chance to socialize. This social component is crucial for mental health, particularly for people who might feel alone because of physical restrictions or a smaller social network.

Chair yoga also encourages independence. It makes everyday actions like reaching for objects, bending, and getting in and out of chairs easier for seniors by strengthening their bodies and increasing their flexibility. A more contented and involved existence can result from this enhanced self-reliance, which can also encourage an active lifestyle and boost confidence.

Safety Procedures and Directives

Even though chair yoga is generally safe for most seniors, caution must be used when doing it. Before beginning any new fitness regimen, it is always advisable to see your doctor, particularly if you have any underlying medical ailments like osteoporosis, heart disease, or joint issues.

Select a supportive chair that is solid and without wheels. Make sure you have enough room to stretch out without running into any walls or furniture. If you experience any pain or discomfort, stop right away and evaluate how you are moving. Gentle, restorative chair yoga should not feel taxing or uncomfortable.

Moreover, pay attention to your breathing. In chair yoga, proper breathing methods are essential for both oxygenating the body and keeping a constant rhythm throughout the exercise. In every pose, try not to hold your breath, and take breaks as needed.

For seniors over 60, chair yoga can be a life-changing practice that improves their physical and mental well-being as long as they follow certain safety precautions. It offers a pleasurable and long-lasting approach to maintain an active lifestyle, gain confidence, and enhance general well-being.

2

Getting Chair Yoga Started

Seniors can keep active and preserve their strength, flexibility, and mental clarity by practicing chair yoga. It is made to be usable by people with physical disabilities or restricted movement. But in order to get the most out of chair yoga, you must set up your space and yourself appropriately. This entails choosing the ideal chair, arranging your area for safety and comfort, and learning some fundamental breathing exercises, all of which are essential to improving your yoga practice.

Selecting the Ideal Chair

The chair itself is, of course, the cornerstone of chair yoga. Selecting the appropriate chair for your practice is essential for both comfort and safety. The chair should ideally be solid and stable, devoid of any wheels or swivel mechanisms that would allow it to suddenly shift. A chair that supports your posture better is one with a flat, solid seat as opposed to one that is excessively cushioned.

Another crucial factor is the chair's height. When seated, your knees should be bent to a 90-degree angle and your feet should be flat on the floor. A chair that is too high can make you feel unsteady or uncomfortable, and a chair that is too low can put strain on your hips and knees. While armrests on a chair might provide stability, they shouldn't limit your range of motion. You might wish to utilize an armless chair for some positions so that you can fully extend your range of motion.

Verify if the chair's back provides adequate support. You can support your lower back with a pillow or folded blanket if it's too hard. Before beginning your practice, always test the chair to make sure it meets your needs and is both safe and comfortable.

Setting Up Your Area

After you've chosen the ideal chair, it's time to set up your area. Your practice area should be roomy enough for you to move about comfortably and clutter-free. To ensure that you may extend your arms and legs without running into anything, make sure there is adequate space surrounding the chair. A space that is wide and unobstructed will not only ensure safety but also contribute to the peaceful atmosphere that encourages mindfulness.

Choose a room with plenty of natural light and few distractions, if at all feasible. If you're practicing at home, think about setting up your chair by a window or in a peaceful place away from distractions. Incorporating factors such as soothing music, soft lighting, or essential oils can also contribute to a more tranquil environment, which can help you relax during your practice.

If the chair feels excessively solid, have a small towel or blanket handy for when you need extra support—for example, cushioning for your back or a place to sit. To stay hydrated during your session, it's also a good idea to keep a glass of water close at hand.

Fundamental Breathing Methods

The foundation of all yoga practice is breathing, and chair yoga is no different. You may achieve a sensation of peace and relaxation as well as ease your way through poses by learning some basic breathing techniques.

Diaphragmatic breathing, often known as belly breathing, is the most basic breathing technique utilized in chair yoga. Sit comfortably in your chair and make sure your shoulders are relaxed and your spine is straight. Grasp your abdomen with one hand and your chest with the other. When you take a breath through your nose, concentrate on relaxing your diaphragm and raising your belly without moving your chest. Then, when you feel your tummy drop, let the air gently and fully through your mouth.

This method eases stress and encourages relaxation while also assisting in the body's increased oxygenation. At the beginning of every chair yoga session, spend a few minutes practicing diaphragmatic breathing to help focus your mind and get your body ready for movement.

Ujjayi breathing, also referred to as "ocean breath," is another breathing method that is frequently employed in yoga. To produce a soft "ocean wave" sound, inhale deeply through your nose and exhale through it while slightly tightening your throat at the back. Throughout your practice, this kind of breathing will help you stay focused and in sync.

In addition to enhancing the physical advantages, chair yoga incorporates proper breathing techniques that also assist reduce stress and increase mindfulness. One of the most important aspects of practicing yoga is being able to stay in the present moment.

You may set yourself up for a rewarding and successful chair yoga practice that enhances your physical and mental well-being by selecting the appropriate chair, setting up a calm environment, and being proficient in fundamental breathing methods.

3

Warm-Up Exercises

It's crucial to gradually warm up your body before beginning your chair yoga practice. Warm-up movements lower your chance of injury, increase the efficiency of your yoga practice, and get your muscles and joints ready for action. These warm-up stretches are a secure and soothing method to improve circulation, relieve stress, and ease into your session for seniors over 60. The four efficient warm-up exercises listed below are seated marching, shoulder rolls, wrist and ankle circles, and mild neck stretches.

Light Neck Stretches

Particularly as we get older, the neck tends to hold a lot of strain, which can cause stiffness and discomfort. Mild neck stretches facilitate the release of tension and enhance the neck and shoulders' range of motion.

Sit comfortably in your chair with your shoulders relaxed and your spine straight to start. Bring your ear close to your shoulder as you gradually tilt your head to the right. Take a few deep breaths and hold this position while noticing the strain on the left side of your neck. The stretch should feel easy and soothing; avoid raising your shoulder or exerting too much force. Return to the center and repeat on the left side after a few breaths.

The back of your neck should then be able to stretch as you incline your chin toward your chest. After a few moments of holding this, gently raise your head back into a neutral posture. Lastly, glance over your shoulder and slowly shift your head to the right. Hold the position for a few breaths, then switch to the left and repeat. It is important to perform these motions slowly and deliberately, focusing on any tight or uncomfortable spots.

Rolls of the Shoulders

A quick and easy approach to release tension in the shoulders, upper back, and neck is to perform shoulder rolls. These areas are frequently prone to strain, and this exercise can help improve circulation and alleviate stiffness there.

Sit up straight and place your arms comfortably by your sides to start. Take a big breath in, then slowly raise your shoulders toward your ears in a circular motion as you release the breath. Roll them back to the beginning position, letting your shoulder blades slip down your back. For five to ten repetitions, repeat this exercise, paying attention to maintaining control and smoothness of motion.

Then, change the direction. Elevate your shoulders with a breath, then roll them down and forward with a release. This aids in releasing any tension in the chest and front of the shoulders. Do five more or ten repetitions. Try to time the movement of rolling your shoulders with your breathing to create a pattern that encourages relaxation.

Ankle and Wrist Circles

Ankle and wrist circles work wonders for enhancing joint mobility in places that stiffen up with aging. By improving flexibility and lubricating the joints, these workouts make it simpler to carry out regular tasks.

Raise your right hand in front of you to start, then gradually start rotating your wrist in a circle. Draw precise, tiny circles in a single direction for ten to fifteen seconds, then change course. Keep an eye out for any soreness or stiffness as you walk. Once you have finished using one wrist, transfer to the left and repeat the motion.

Sit back in your chair and elevate your right foot a little bit off the floor to perform ankle circles. With your ankle, point your toes and start slowly rotating in one direction for ten to fifteen seconds before turning around. Reduce the size of the movement if you experience any discomfort. Repeat with the left ankle after completing the right ankle. This exercise increases ankle mobility and improves circulation in the lower legs.

Marching while seated

Marching while seated is an excellent method to increase blood flow, contract your leg muscles, and strengthen your core. Enhances coordination and helps warm up the lower body with this exercise.

With your arms at your sides and your feet flat on the floor, assume a tall seated position. Starting with your back straight, raise your right knee as high as comfortable toward your chest. As though you were marching in place, lower your right foot back to the ground and then raise your left knee in the same manner.

You can raise the speed if it feels comfortable after starting off gently and concentrating on keeping proper posture and controlled motions.

Swing your opposing arm forward with each knee lift for improved coordination, much like you would when you walk. Try to complete 10–20 reps on each leg, or until your muscles are sufficiently warmed up.

In summary

You must warm up your body for chair yoga with these movements: seated marching, shoulder rolls, wrist and ankle circles, and moderate neck stretches. They assist foster a relaxed and concentrated mindset for the practice that lies ahead while enhancing flexibility, circulation, and injury prevention. These warm-ups will help you lay a strong foundation for a secure and productive chair yoga practice.

4

Seated Yoga Poses

In spite of their limited mobility, elders can still benefit from yoga with chair yoga's gentle and safe approach. With the chair's support, seated yoga poses can increase muscular strength, encourage relaxation, and improve flexibility. Sitting Mountain Pose, Seated Forward Bend, Seated Twist, Seated Side Stretch, and Seated Cat-Cow Stretch are five beneficial sitting yoga positions that are perfect for seniors.

seated mountain position

The foundation for many other sitting yoga postures, sitting Mountain Pose is a great method to enhance your body awareness, posture, and concentration. It promotes a sense of solidity and grounding while assisting with spinal alignment.

Start by sitting up straight in your chair and placing your feet hip-width apart on the floor. Put your hands on your thighs or at your sides, palms down, and contract your core muscles to support your spine. To open up your chest, rotate your shoulders slightly back and down while maintaining a straight back.

While maintaining this position, visualize a string drawing your head's crown upward, elongating your spine. Breathe deeply many times, allowing your body to become solid and balanced. This posture lays a solid foundation for the rest of your practice by assisting you in developing body awareness and mindfulness.

Forward Bend Seating

A mild stretch that works the hips, hamstrings, and lower back is the seated forward bend. It encourages relaxation and aids in the release of spinal tension.

Place your feet level on the floor and start by sitting at the edge of your chair. Take a deep breath to stretch your spine. Then, slowly tilt forward from your hips and extend your hands toward the floor or your feet. Fold forward, allowing your neck to stretch and your head to relax.

Don't force the stretch; if you are unable to reach the floor, just place your hands on your shins or knees. The idea is not to round your spine but to maintain a long back. Feel the stretch in your legs and back as you hold this position for a few breaths. Using your core, carefully roll back up to a seated posture while taking a breath to exit the pose.

Twist when sitting

The Seated Twist is a great pose to increase internal organ massage and spinal motion, which can help with digestion. Additionally, it eases shoulder and back stress.

With your hands resting on your thighs and your feet flat on the floor, take a tall stance on your chair. Lengthen your spine by inhaling, and then slowly twist your torso to the right while supporting yourself with your left hand on your right leg. You can put your right hand on the chair's back. Maintain a long spine and don't force the twist; instead, allow your body to flow in sync with your breathing.

Feel the stretch in your torso and vertebrae as you hold the twist for a few breaths. After taking a breath, carefully bring yourself back to the center and repeat the twist on the left side. This pose helps release tension in the upper body and promotes spinal flexibility.

Side Stretch While Seated

Seated Side Stretches work on the lower back, rib cage, and sides of the body. It opens up the chest to facilitate deep breathing and increases spinal flexibility.

To begin, take a tall seat in your chair and place your feet flat on the ground. Taking a breath, extend your right arm through your fingertips and elevate it overhead. Stretch your right side and slowly lean to the left as you release the breath. Avoid bringing your chest down by keeping your left hand supported by your thigh or chair. Feel your spine lengthening and your rib cage expanding as you hold the stretch for a few deep breaths.

After taking a breath to get back to the middle, extend your left side again. Deep, full breaths are easier to take in this position because it opens up the chest and helps the spine become more flexible.

Cat-Cow Stretch in Sitting

A dynamic exercise that strengthens the core, increases spinal flexibility, and eases back strain is the seated cat-cow stretch. This flow is a great way to encourage both relaxation and mobility.

Place your feet level on the floor and start by sitting at the edge of your chair. Grasp your knees with your hands. The "Cow" position is achieved by arching your back, elevating your chest, and tilting your pelvis forward while you inhale. Stretch the front of your body and open your chest slightly as you cast a glance upward.

The "Cat" position is achieved by rounding your back, tucking your chin into your chest, and drawing your belly button in toward your spine as you release the breath. Your upper back will feel a light stretch as your shoulders come forward.

With every breath, keep switching between these two positions: exhale as you round into Cat and inhale as you arch into Cow. Continue in this manner for a few cycles while moving slowly and deliberately. This stretch helps release tension in the shoulders and lower back and enhances spinal mobility.

In summary

Seniors can increase their flexibility, strength, and general well-being with these simple yet powerful seated yoga poses: Seated Mountain Pose, Seated Forward Bend, Seated Twist, Seated Side Stretch, and Seated Cat-Cow Stretch. Regularly achieving these positions can improve mental and physical well-being and lead to a more contented and balanced way of living.

5

Strengthening Exercises

Not only does chair yoga help with flexibility and stretching, but it's also a terrific technique for seniors to safely and easily gain strength. Exercises for strengthening the muscles aid in maintaining muscle mass, enhancing balance, and supporting the functional motions required for daily tasks. For senior citizens doing chair yoga, try these five efficient strengthening exercises: Seated Knee Extensions, Seated Side Leg Raises, Chair Pose with Arm Lift, and Seated Arm Presses.

Leg Lifts While Seated

Leg lifts while seated are a great way to develop your lower body, especially your hip flexors and quads. For tasks like walking, getting out of a chair, and ascending stairs, these muscles are necessary.

With your feet flat on the floor, sit up straight to complete Seated Leg Lifts. For support, rest your hands on the chair's sides. Taking a breath, raise your right leg off the ground while maintaining a straight leg position. Lift by using your thigh and core muscles, trying to lift the leg as high as feels comfortable. After a few seconds of holding the raise, carefully and slowly lower the leg.

With the same level of concentration, raise and drop the leg as you did on the left side. On each side, perform ten to fifteen repetitions, or however many feels comfortable. This exercise increases stability and strengthens the leg muscles, which can help reduce the risk of falling and increase mobility.

Arms raised in the chair pose

Chair Pose with Arm Lift is an effective full-body workout that enhances posture and balance while strengthening the arms, legs, and core. It is similar to the standard yoga Chair Pose, but it makes use of the chair itself as support.

With your feet level on the floor and hip-width apart, take a seat at the edge of your chair to begin. Take a long breath in, and as you release it, push through your feet to elevate your lower body off the chair just a little bit so that it appears to be hovering over the seat. Raise your arms upwards while maintaining a comfortable posture in your shoulders. To stabilize your spine, contract your core, and take a few deep breaths to maintain the position.

Try to hold the hover for a longer period of time—five to ten seconds—to up the challenge. After lowering yourself back to the chair gradually, repeat the motion eight to twelve times. This pose works the upper body and core to improve general stability while strengthening the legs and glutes.

Extensions of the Knee While Seated

Strengthening the quadriceps, which are essential for leg strength and knee stability, may be achieved with ease by performing Seated Knee Extensions. For seniors who need to strengthen their knees to increase their mobility, this activity is excellent.

Place your feet firmly on the floor and sit up straight in your chair to start. For support, hold on to the chair's sides. After taking a deep breath, extend your right leg by lifting your foot off the ground and straightening it until it reaches your full length. Maintain your foot flexed and your thigh engaged.

After a few seconds of holding the extension, softly drop your leg such that your foot touches the floor again. On the left side, repeat. Do ten to fifteen repetitions on each leg. The muscles surrounding the knee joint are strengthened by this exercise, which is essential for preserving leg strength and enabling daily activities like standing and walking.

Side Leg Raises While Seated

The muscles in the hips and outer thighs, which are crucial for balance and lateral movement, are strengthened with side leg raises while seated. Additionally, this exercise can help increase hip flexibility and mobility.

Place your feet flat on the floor and take a seat at the edge of your chair to begin. For support, hold on to the chair's sides. Breathe in, and as you release, extend your right leg as far to the side as feels comfortable while maintaining a straight leg and flexed foot. To keep your body stable when you lift, contract your thigh and core muscles.

After a few seconds of holding the lift, carefully return your leg to its initial position. Repeat on the left side, carefully raising and lowering the leg. Do ten to twelve repetitions on each side. Targeting the hips and thighs, seated side leg raises enhance lower body strength and balance, two factors crucial to avoiding falls and preserving mobility.

Arm Presses While Seated

Using only your body weight, seated arm presses are an easy method to strengthen the arms, shoulders, and chest. Building upper body strength is a prerequisite for tasks like pushing, carrying, and lifting. This workout helps achieve this goal.

With your feet flat on the ground, take a straight seat in your chair. Put your hands together at a height that allows your palms to touch at the chest. Take a deep breath in, then contract your chest and arm muscles by pressing your hands together as you exhale. Press and hold for five to ten seconds, then let go.

You can push your hands together and extend your arms straight in front of you or overhead for more intensity. Press again ten or twelve times. Particularly for seniors who might have restricted shoulder or arm mobility, seated arm presses are a great approach to strengthen the upper body.

In summary

The following strengthening exercises are great for increasing muscle strength, balance, and mobility: Seated Leg Lifts, Chair Pose with Arm Lift, Seated Knee Extensions, Seated Side Leg Raises, and Seated Arm Presses. Seniors' general quality of life can be enhanced, their independence can be maintained, and falls can be avoided with regular practice of these activities. Including these poses in your chair yoga practice offers a comprehensive approach to mental and physical health.

6

Flexibility and Balance

Particularly for seniors, flexibility and balance are critical elements of general fitness. They facilitate mobility, lower the chance of falling, and improve one's capacity to carry out everyday duties with assurance. With slow, deliberate movements and gentle stretches, chair yoga provides a secure and efficient method to enhance balance and flexibility. The following are some essential activities that can be beneficial: chair balance exercises, seated torso twists, seated hamstring stretches, and seated calf stretches.

Stretching Your Hamstrings While Seated

The hamstrings, which are found at the back of the thighs, are the focus of the easy-to-do but effective Seated Hamstring Stretch. Strong hamstrings can reduce lower back pain and increase leg mobility, which facilitates standing and walking.

Place your feet flat on the floor and sit at the edge of your chair to perform the Seated Hamstring Stretch. With your toes pointed upward and your heel flat on the ground, extend your right leg straight out in front of you. Breathe deeply in, then release the air as you slowly bend forward from your hips and reach for your ankle or toes. When reaching, maintain a straight back and refrain from bending your spine.

Your thigh should feel somewhat stretched in the back. While you hold the stretch for 15 to 20 seconds, take slow breaths and let your muscles release tension. On an inhale, return to an upright position and repeat with your left leg. This stretch promotes improved posture and increases leg flexibility.

Stretching Your Calf While Seated

One useful exercise for improving lower limb flexibility is the Seated Calf Stretch, which targets the hamstrings and calves in particular. Calf muscles that are flexible are essential for stability and balance because they facilitate standing and walking.

First, take a straight seat on your chair and place both of your feet flat on the ground. With your heel flat on the ground, extend your right leg in front of you. Your toes should point upward when you flex your foot. Take a long breath in, and as you release it, gently bring your toes back toward your body with your hands, a towel, or a yoga strap if you can.

Feel the back of your lower thigh and your calf muscle lengthening as you hold the stretch for 15 to 20 seconds. After taking a deep breath, gradually release the stretch. On the left leg, repeat. This stretch helps avoid leg cramps and stiffness in addition to increasing flexibility.

Exercises for Chair Balance

Chair Balance Exercises: As we age, maintaining our independence and minimizing falls need improved stability and coordination. Seniors can safely perform these exercises by sitting or utilizing a chair for support.

Sitting at the edge of your chair with your feet flat on the ground is a basic balance exercise. For support, grasp the chair's sides. Take a deep breath, and as you release it, raise your right foot a few inches off the ground. Use your core to stay balanced. After holding the posture for five to ten seconds, bring your foot back down. With your left foot, repeat.

You might try raising one arm and your foot simultaneously to make it more difficult. This strengthens your upper body and core, improving your overall stability. Work out 8–10 times on each side. Exercises for Chair Balance develop the muscles involved in balance, which is necessary for daily tasks including walking, turning, and reaching.

Twists of the Torso when Seated

One excellent technique to increase spine flexibility and enhance upper body mobility is to perform seated torso twists. In addition to helping to improve posture and promote deeper breathing, twisting motions also stretch the muscles along the sides of the torso.

Sit up straight in your chair and place your feet flat on the floor to perform Seated Torso Twists. For support, rest your hands on your knees. As you exhale, gently twist your torso to the right, supporting yourself with your left hand on your right knee. This will stretch your spine. Remain upright and refrain from exerting force on the twist. Feel the stretch in your torso and vertebrae as you hold the twist for a few breaths.

Upon coming back to the center, take a breath and proceed with the left twist, positioning your right hand on your left knee. Repeat this twist five to eight times on each side. Seated torso twists promote improved digestion and circulation while also increasing spinal flexibility.

In summary

Enhance your mobility, stability, and general well-being by adding balancing and flexibility exercises to your chair yoga practice. Gentle yet efficient methods to improve flexibility and balance include chair balance exercises, seated hamstring stretches, seated calf stretches, and seated torso twists. Seniors who regularly perform these motions can increase their mobility with ease and confidence, preserve their independence, and lower their risk of falling. These exercises can help you live a more pain-free, healthy, and active existence with regular effort.

7

Relaxation Techniques

Any workout regimen must include relaxation, but chair yoga for seniors in particular needs it even more. Relaxation not only eases mental tension but also eases physical tension, decreases blood pressure, and enhances general wellbeing. Many simple relaxation techniques that are beneficial for both physical and mental well-being are provided by chair yoga. These consist of Progressive Muscle Relaxation, Gentle Breathing Exercises, Guided Visualization, and Seated Meditation.

Meditation in Chairs

One of the easiest yet most powerful methods of relaxing is sitting meditation. It eases mental tension, boosts focus, and quiets the mind. Seniors who may have mobility issues can safely and conveniently practice seated meditation in the comfort of their own chair.

Place your hands softly on your lap and sit comfortably in your chair with your feet flat on the floor. Shut your eyes and inhale deeply through your nose. Let go of any tension in your body by gently exhaling through your mouth. Pay attention to your breathing and the feeling of air coming into and going out of your body.

Bring your focus back to your breathing softly and without passing judgment if your thoughts stray. You can practice for five minutes at first, and then as you get more comfortable, you can practice for longer periods of time. Frequent meditation practice can result in increased inner calm, less anxiety, and better mental clarity.

Assisted Visualization

Using the imagination to conjure up serene and tranquil mental images is the basis of the effective relaxation technique known as guided visualization. By shifting the mind from problems to peaceful, pleasant ideas, this technique helps lower stress and fosters a sense of serenity.

Close your eyes and get into a comfortable chair to begin practicing guided visualization. Start by relaxing your body with a few deep breaths. Next, picture yourself in a serene, lovely setting, such as a beach, forest, or garden. To help you imagine the sight, use all of your senses: smell the fresh air, see the brilliant colors all around you, and hear the noises of nature.

Allow all of your anxiety and stress to dissolve as you lose yourself in this mental image. Take a few minutes to enjoy your serene surroundings and give yourself permission to be at ease. When you're ready, carefully return your focus to the here and now. Breathe deeply a few times before opening your eyes.

With the aid of guided visualization, one can feel happier, more at ease, and more relaxed. It's a simple method that may be used at any time, although it works best right before bed or in stressful situations.

Easy Breathing Techniques

In chair yoga, the foundation of relaxation is the practice of gentle breathing exercises. The relaxation response in the body is triggered by these exercises, which concentrate on deepening and slowing down the breath. Breathing exercises assist in lowering blood pressure, lowering stress levels, and enhancing brain oxygen flow.

The 4-7-8 technique is one easy breathing technique. Sit up straight in your chair and place your hands on your lap to start. Take four slow, deep breaths through your nose. After holding your breath for seven counts, let out all of it through your mouth for eight counts, whooshing as you go.

This cycle should be repeated four times, or as often as is comfortable. This method aids in heart rate reduction, nervous system calmness, and relaxation. Any time of day is a good opportunity to practice breathing techniques, but they work best right before bed or during stressful situations to assist encourage peaceful sleep.

Gradual Relaxation of the Muscles

To relieve physical tension and encourage relaxation, progressive muscle relaxation, or PMR, is a technique that entails tensing and then relaxing various muscle groups. Because this exercise is done while seated, it's ideal for elders who do chair yoga.

Place your feet flat on the floor while sitting comfortably in your chair to begin practicing PMR. Start by tensing your foot muscles by curling your toes and maintaining the tension for a few seconds to a minute. Then, relax and pay attention to how your feet feel as they become lighter.

Ascend your body, starting with your calves and working your way up to your thighs. Give each muscle a brief period of tenseness, then release it. Your shoulders, neck, and face should all feel extremely relaxed by the time you get there. Progressive muscular relaxation can even lessen stiffness or pain in the muscles by releasing stored tension and lowering stress.

In summary

Adding relaxation methods to your chair yoga practice will help you feel better both physically and mentally. Progressive muscle relaxation eases physical stress, gentle breathing exercises create calmness through focused breathing, guided visualization promotes tranquil mental imagery, and seated meditation helps calm the mind. These methods are ideal for seniors who want to improve their general health and quality of life since they are easy to use, affordable, and very effective at fostering relaxation and lowering stress. Frequent use of these relaxation techniques can result in long-term advantages like deeper inner peace, greater sleep, and decreased anxiety.

8

Creating a Routine

Seniors might experience significant improvements in their physical and mental health by establishing a regular chair yoga practice. Over time, seniors can enhance their flexibility, strength, balance, and relaxation by establishing a disciplined routine. This part will cover how to include chair yoga with other exercises, establish attainable objectives to monitor your progress, and create a daily chair yoga practice.

How to Start a Chair Yoga Practice Every Day

Consistency is essential for developing any new habit or skill. Creating a regular chair yoga practice is a great way to reap long-term advantages like improved mobility, stress reduction, and improved balance. Seniors might begin with a modest exercise regimen and progressively increase it, enabling their bodies to adjust and become more resilient over time.

Select the time of day that is most convenient for you to start. Some people find that doing yoga in the morning gives them energy for the day, while others might prefer an evening practice to relax before bed. Even just ten to fifteen minutes a day can have a big impact, especially for newcomers. You can progressively extend the length of your practice as you get more accustomed to the exercises.

Warm-up stretches and mild breathing techniques are a good way to ease into your daily routine. Concentrate on adopting stances that suit your body's needs and feel comfortable. Because chair yoga allows for changes, you can change up the poses to suit any discomfort or physical limits. Recall that consistency, not intensity, is the secret to success. Positive outcomes can be achieved over time with even a little, mild practice every day.

Chair Yoga in Combination with Other Exercises

Even while chair yoga provides a thorough workout for relaxation, strength, and flexibility, incorporating it with other workouts can result in a more well-rounded fitness regimen. A well-rounded fitness regimen for seniors may incorporate strength training, flexibility training, and aerobic exercise.

You might want to include low-impact exercises like swimming, cycling, or walking in your weekly schedule. These aerobic and endurance-boosting activities are a great supplement to chair yoga. Specifically, walking is an excellent means of preserving joint mobility and heart health.

An additional beneficial supplement to your exercise regimen is strength training. Resistance bands, light weights, and even common household items like water bottles can be used for exercises that target and improve your arms, legs, and core. Chair yoga activities assist improved posture, balance, and overall mobility through stronger muscles.

Chair yoga along with these other activities can help you maintain your strength, flexibility, and cardiovascular health in a comprehensive way. Remember to listen to your body and exercise caution not to overdo it. Take breaks when needed and allow yourself to recuperate in between more demanding activities.

Creating sensible objectives and monitoring advancement

Setting and monitoring attainable objectives and monitoring your progress is one of the best strategies to maintain motivation during any exercise program. Setting attainable objectives will help you feel accomplished and motivate you to continue practicing chair yoga, regardless of how long you've been doing it.

Decide at the outset what you want to get out of chair yoga. Which would you prefer—more relaxation, less discomfort, better balance, or improved flexibility? Your objectives ought to take into account your unique wants and skills. For instance, over the course of a month, you might try to maintain a seated yoga pose longer or extend your practice time from 10 to 20 minutes.

Keeping a journal of your daily practice might be an easy way to monitor your development. Note the activities you do, the amount of time you spent practicing, and your pre- and post-exercise feelings. You might also want to record any gains you have in strength, flexibility, or mood. You'll be able to gauge your progress over time and identify any areas that still require work.

A fitness or health professional you work with can also help you set objectives and monitor your progress. Rewarding yourself for little victories along the way can help you maintain your chair yoga practice and gain confidence.

In summary

Developing a daily practice, incorporating it with other types of exercise, and establishing realistic goals are all part of creating a chair yoga regimen. The secret to enjoying chair yoga's long-term advantages is consistency, and adding in other exercises like strength training or walking makes for a more comprehensive fitness routine. Setting attainable objectives and monitoring your development will help you maintain motivation as you gradually improve your flexibility, balance, and general health. A well-designed chair yoga program can offer elders a secure and efficient means of preserving their physical and emotional health.

9

Adapting Chair Yoga for Specific Needs

Chair yoga is a very adaptable type of exercise that has several advantages for seniors and people with varying physical capacities. Its adaptability to persons with different levels of movement and unique health concerns, such as arthritis, is one of its greatest features. This section will cover chair yoga for arthritis, mobility changes, and adapting practices for wheelchair users.

Adjustments for Limited Mobility

It's critical to adapt chair yoga for seniors with restricted mobility in order to assure their comfort and safety. With these adjustments, people can take part in their practice to the fullest without placing unnecessary physical pressure on their bodies.

First things first: select a strong chair that offers enough support; ideally, it should be wheel-free and equipped with armrests if necessary. Reducing pressure on the knees and hips when sitting and standing can be facilitated by a chair with an elevated seat. Additional comfort and support can be added by tucking a cushion under the thighs or behind the back.

You may adjust many chair yoga positions by lowering the intensity or range of motion. Those with restricted flexibility, for instance, can place their hands on their thighs during the Seated Forward Bend instead of reaching for their feet. In a similar vein, muscles can still be efficiently engaged during Seated Leg Lifts by raising the leg only a few inches off the floor as opposed to fully extending it.

It's critical to keep in mind that even modest actions can have a significant impact. Working within one's boundaries rather than pushing past discomfort is the aim. Strength, flexibility, and mobility can all be gradually increased with time.

Yoga in Chairs for Arthritis

Seniors with arthritis frequently experience joint pain, stiffness, and inflammation. For those who have arthritis, chair yoga is a great form of exercise since it offers soft, low-impact movement that supports joint health without aggravating existing discomfort.

The secret to chair yoga for arthritis sufferers is to concentrate on slow, deliberate movements that promote joint mobility and ease stiffness. Shoulder rolls and wrist and ankle circles are great warm-up movements that help loosen up the joints and get the body ready for more difficult positions. Stretching gently, such as the Seated Side Stretch, helps to release tension in the muscles that surround the joints and promote flexibility.

It's crucial to avoid maintaining positions for extended periods of time or exerting excessive force during stretches for those with arthritis. To avoid straining the joints, movements should be moderate and deliberate, letting the body move naturally. It's preferable to stop and either adjust the stance or try an alternative one if any movement causes pain.

Apart from its physical advantages, chair yoga can aid in pain management through the promotion of relaxation and reduction of tension, both of which are known to worsen the symptoms of arthritis. The mind can be calmed and discomfort can be relieved by breathing techniques and meditation.

Modifying Pose for People in Wheelchairs

Wheelchair users can safely and effectively maintain strength, flexibility, and balance with chair yoga, which eliminates the need to stand or alternate between poses. Wheelchair users can participate in a full chair yoga session with the appropriate modifications.

Many classic yoga postures can be modified to accommodate a seated position when practicing chair yoga in a wheelchair. For instance, you can perform the Seated Cat-Cow Stretch, which involves rounding and arching your back, by gripping the armrests of your wheelchair. Without putting undue weight on the lower body, this opens the chest and stretches the spine.

Additionally, wheelchair users can concentrate on strengthening exercises and stretches for the upper body. For example, seated arm presses work the arms and shoulders, while seated forward bends, with the feet still on the footrest, provide a mild stretch for the legs and back.

Pose variations like Seated Twists help with flexibility and balance, enhancing core strength, and preserving a healthy range of motion in the torso. Incorporating breathing exercises like the 4-7-8 technique will also help you relax and get the most out of your yoga practice.

Wheelchair users may occasionally choose to enlist the help of a caregiver or yoga instructor, particularly when attempting new positions or motions. It's crucial to make sure that every action is secure and pleasant, avoiding any workouts that could overwork the body.

In summary

People with restricted mobility, arthritis, or those in wheelchairs can benefit from chair yoga's modifications without experiencing any discomfort or risk of harm. Chair yoga can be adjusted to accommodate a range of physical capacities by changing up the postures, emphasizing joint-friendly activities, and adding flexibility and balance practice. Regardless of one's physical condition, chair yoga is a great practice for boosting joint health, relaxation, and overall well-being because of its gentle and adjustable nature.

<u>10</u>

Success Stories and Testimonials

Many seniors' lives have been changed by chair yoga, which provides an easily accessible, low-impact method of enhancing both physical and emotional well-being. Seniors' overall quality of life has increased, their mobility has been restored, and their discomfort has decreased because of this gentle therapy. This section will offer expert views and advice that showcase the advantages of chair yoga, along with an exploration of some heartwarming success stories from seniors who practice the pose.

Motivational Narratives from Elderly Chair Yoga Practitioners

Mary, 72, Overcomes Severe Illness:

Osteoarthritis caused Mary, a 72-year-old retiree, to suffer from persistent pain in her hips and knees. She gave up on physical activity completely since she found traditional workout routines to be too unpleasant. She made the decision to attempt chair yoga after learning about it from a friend.

Mary was apprehensive at first, thinking the movements would exacerbate her discomfort. Nevertheless, she started with basic stretches and breathing techniques with the assistance of a nearby chair yoga instructor. Her discomfort gradually lessened, and she began to notice that her joints were less stiff in the mornings. She started going to lessons frequently and worked her way up to more difficult postures like Seated Forward Bends and Leg Lifts.

Mary has discovered a new sense of freedom and now does chair yoga five times a week. Her range of motion has greatly increased, and she no longer experiences everyday discomfort.

"Chair yoga has given me back my independence," Mary explains. "I can move freely again without worrying about pain."

John, 78, Finding His Calm and Self-Belief Back:

Following a hip injury sustained in a fall, John, 78, noticed that he was less inclined to move around than before. He lost all trust in his ability to walk and perform daily tasks. Chair yoga was suggested by his physical therapist as a component of his rehabilitation, specifically for the purpose of regaining strength and balance.

John attempted chair yoga in the hopes of strengthening his stability, despite his initial skepticism. John gradually regained his strength and balance using chair balance exercises and poses like Seated Side Leg Raises and Torso Twists. He was no longer afraid of falling because he could feel his muscles moving.

After six months of training, John is once again able to stroll around his house with assurance and even goes for quick walks outside. "Chair yoga helped me get back on my feet, both literally and figuratively," John shares. "It's given me the confidence to live my life fully again."

Anna, eighty-one, Reducing Anxiety and Stress:

At eighty-one, Anna was experiencing more and more worry as a result of the COVID-19 pandemic's isolation and unpredictability. She often went to bed without feeling sleepy, and she was always worried. Her daughter recommended chair yoga as a stress-reduction technique.

Anna added gentle breathing exercises and seated meditation to her daily regimen because she found comfort in these peaceful techniques. Her anxiousness significantly decreased once she started doing yoga for just ten minutes a day. She had better quality sleep, and she felt more centered all day. "Chair yoga gave me peace of mind when everything around me felt chaotic," Anna explains. "It's my daily source of calm."

Professional Opinions and Suggestions

Healthcare specialists and fitness experts have come to recognize chair yoga for its many health benefits and accessibility, especially for senior citizens. Experts concur that practicing chair yoga can help older persons keep or regain their physical health in a safe and effective manner while also fostering their mental and emotional wellbeing.

Specialist in Geriatrics, Dr. Susan Miller:

For seniors who may have limited mobility or who are managing chronic diseases like osteoporosis or arthritis, chair yoga is a great form of exercise. According to geriatric specialist Dr. Susan Miller, "it offers a low-impact way to improve flexibility, balance, and muscle strength without putting strain on the joints." "The breathing and relaxation techniques used in chair yoga also help to reduce stress and anxiety, which is crucial for maintaining mental health as we age."

Lisa Martinez, Senior Yoga Teacher Certification:

"One of the best things about chair yoga is that it can be done by anyone, no matter what their physical limitations are," says Lisa Martinez, a yoga instructor with certification who specializes in senior wellness. "I've worked with people in their 80s and 90s who have had incredible gains in their quality of life and mobility. The secret is to increase your practice gradually, pay attention to your body, and start out cautiously."

Both experts stress that the goal of chair yoga is to foster a holistic sense of well-being in addition to physical activity. Prior to beginning chair yoga, they advise seniors to speak with their healthcare professional, particularly if they have any pre-existing illnesses. They also advise seniors to work with a trained instructor to guarantee appropriate technique and adaptations.

In summary

The positive outcomes of senior citizens like Mary, John, and Anna provide evidence of chair yoga's transformational potential. Chair yoga provides an accessible route to improved health and wellness, ranging from lowering anxiety and chronic pain to enhancing confidence and balance. Expert opinions support the notion that chair yoga is a flexible, safe, and beneficial form of exercise for seniors that offers mental and physical health advantages. Chair yoga can be an incredibly effective technique for improving your quality of life, whether your goals are to stay active, restore mobility, or lower your stress level.

WORKBOOK

Chapter 1: Introduction

Exercises and Reflections:

1. **Reflect on Your Current Exercise Routine:**
   - How does your current exercise routine (if any) affect your overall well-being? What challenges do you face in maintaining it?
2. **Identify Personal Goals:**
   - What are your primary goals for practicing chair yoga? (e.g., improving flexibility, reducing pain, enhancing relaxation)

Chapter 2: Getting Started with Chair Yoga

Exercises and Reflections:

1. **Evaluate Your Chair:**
    o   Describe the chair you plan to use
        for chair yoga. How does it meet
        the requirements for a safe and
        comfortable practice?
2. **Create Your Yoga Space:**
    o   How will you prepare your space
        for chair yoga? List any
        adjustments or additions you need
        to make to ensure a supportive
        environment.

Chapter 3: Warm-Up Exercises

Exercises and Reflections:

1. **Warm-Up Routine Assessment:**
   - Practice the warm-up exercises outlined. How do you feel before and after performing these exercises? Are there any areas where you feel particularly tense?
2. **Modify for Comfort:**
   - If you experience discomfort during any warm-up exercise, what modifications can you make to improve comfort while still benefiting from the exercise?

Chapter 4: Seated Yoga Poses

Exercises and Reflections:

1. **Pose Practice Log:**
   - Try each seated yoga pose described. Which poses felt most comfortable and which were challenging? Record your observations and any adjustments you made.
2. **Pose Benefits Analysis:**
   - Reflect on the benefits you experienced from the seated yoga poses. How have these poses impacted your flexibility, balance, and overall sense of well-being?

Chapter 5: Strengthening Exercises

Exercises and Reflections:

1. **Strength Assessment:**
   - Complete the strengthening exercises listed. How did each exercise impact your muscle strength and endurance? Did you notice any improvement in your ability to perform daily activities?
2. **Adjusting Intensity:**
   - If you found any strengthening exercise too difficult, how did you modify it? How do you plan to gradually increase the intensity as you build strength?

Chapter 6: Flexibility and Balance

Exercises and Reflections:

1. **Flexibility Evaluation:**
   - Perform the flexibility and balance exercises provided. How do you assess your current level of flexibility and balance? Were there any noticeable improvements after practicing?
2. **Balance Challenges:**
   - Identify any specific challenges you faced while performing balance exercises. What strategies can you use to improve your balance in these areas?

Chapter 7: Relaxation Techniques

Exercises and Reflections:

1. **Relaxation Technique Experience:**
   - Practice each relaxation technique outlined. Which technique did you find most effective in reducing stress and promoting relaxation? Describe your experience.
2. **Daily Integration Plan:**
   - How can you integrate these relaxation techniques into your daily routine? Create a plan for incorporating at least one technique into your day regularly.

Chapter 8: Creating a Routine

Exercises and Reflections:

1. **Routine Development:**
    - Outline a chair yoga routine that fits into your daily schedule. How will you ensure consistency and adapt your routine as needed?
2. **Goal Setting and Tracking:**
    - Set realistic goals for your chair yoga practice. How will you track your progress towards these goals? What methods will you use to evaluate and adjust your practice over time?

Chapter 9: Adapting Chair Yoga for Specific Needs

Exercises and Reflections:

1. **Modification Assessment:**
   - Reflect on any specific needs or limitations you have. How will you adapt chair yoga poses to accommodate these needs? Record any modifications you plan to make.
2. **Adaptive Techniques Journal:**
   - After practicing the adapted chair yoga poses, how do you feel about the effectiveness of these modifications? What other adaptations might you need to try?

A Special Gift For

The Reader

HERE IS THE BONUS VIDEO, I PROMISE TO GIVE YOU.

TITLE: **10 Minute Chair Yoga for Seniors, Beginners**

SCAN THIS QR CODE TO WATCH THIS VIDEO NOW